LIVING A FULL LIFE
WITH
CONGESTIVE HEART
FAILURE.

By Sally Pederson

D1409930

Thank you for purchasing this book. Please review
this book on Amazon. I need your feedback so I can
make the next version even better. Thank you very
much.

For other books by this author go to:
https://www.amazon.com/author/sallypederson

Table of Contents –

Introduction

'My heart beats for you' – for an individual who speaks these words nothing could be farther from the truth. This is because our heart beats first to ensure our existence and only then it could beat for anyone else. Such is the importance of this internal organ that its rhythmic beating is the very essence of existence – a heart that beats is a symbol of life while one that may have stopped beating is indicative of a life snuffed out. There are many reasons leading to the latter and one of the most insidious as also the least discussed is a medical condition known as congestive heart failure.

When the heart is deprived of the requisite amount of oxygen needed to carry out normal functioning, it feels congested and if ignored, this is the condition that will eventually lead to congestive heart failure. Many times it is the aftermath of an already existing cardiac condition and the prognosis often depends on the seriousness of the initial state. Therefore, doctors specialized in the field, namely cardiologists, often emphasize on prevention rather than cure as an effective way to avert its incidence. With existing therapies and new revolutionary developments like stem cell research and translational research, chances of recovery have also significantly improved.

In-depth study into this arena has also made evident the fact that stemming the problem in its nascent stages by affecting lifestyle changes is one of the most effective ways of nipping it in the bud. The most common, also strongly recommended mantra, preaches a combination of healthy diet, exercise and wearing loose clothes that do not hinder blood flow in any manner. True though it might be that these are difficult to promulgate on a daily basis, following these strictures as closely as possible does have a positive impact.

Ultimately, considering the fact that every human being has a heart and hence is susceptible to congestive heart failure, this condition should be one of the major concerns of agencies responsible for public health. One of the noteworthy names in this regard is that of American Medical Association but equally shocking is the lack of comprehensive data which should be compiled by other involved organizations. While it is commendable that doctors do everything within their capability to truncate this killer condition, the organizational support that they should be receiving is negligible. There are only a small percentage of hospitals on a nationwide scale that are adequately equipped to deal with this problem and provide post-surgical care.

Finally, the onus is on the Government to take initiative and allocate adequate resources so that it can be addressed on a nation-wide scale and that victims diagnosed with it can look forward to a happy and trouble-free future instead of losing hope.

The Heart

"I love you with all my heart" or "My heart is broken". How many times to we hear words like these? Every day the heart is used metaphorically to describe love and pain. This is a part of who we are as humans, the other being having a healthy, vital heart.

Although the heart is entwined with our emotions, it is a real and integral part of our body and its primary function is to keep us alive and healthy. The health of the heart can be measured by taking blood pressure and the results provide the first indication of any possible problems that may be in occurring. There are two parts to reading blood pressure - systolic and diastolic pressure. Of these, the former measures the strength with which the left ventricle is contracting, meaning any problem in pumping blood would cause systolic heart failure. Likewise, when the left ventricle is unable to relax or fill completely then diastolic heart failure occurs. A healthy heart needs to beat with vigor and relax enough to be refilled with blood.

There are a number of factors that contribute towards having a healthy heart. According to the American Heart Association, the Cleveland Clinic and other medical centers, caring for your heart entails paying attention to aspects like stress, lifestyle, exercise and diet to name a few.

A very important part of maintaining a healthy heart by reducing stress is exercise and it is not necessarily limited only to gym or gym equipment. It is possible to incorporate certain simple exercises in the daily routine and performing these for even 20 minutes a day would go a long way towards helping your heart. To start, sit in a comfortable chair in loose clothes and start by rotating your feet and ankles till you feel the strain. Next, raise your legs and hold them for about five minutes followed by hands and arms, one at a time. Finally, move your head up and down and then back and forth.

Another important aspect of heart health is a proper diet plan. More important than what you eat, is how much you eat and how often. That said it is still advisable to stay away from foods like fats and sugars that are commonly labeled as being unhealthy.

The sad truth is that heart disease is the nations' leading cause of death, and yet there is only scattered and incomplete data on it. While the American Heart Association has put together some pertinent information, much to its disappointment the U.S. Government has made no attempt to collaborate in this effort. While it is true that we think of the heart only in terms of love and hate, we eventually have to start looking at the real heart in terms of arteries and veins and realize the effect on our heart by doing the things we do.

Ultimately, we can take heart in the knowledge that our heart cares for us for as long as we care for it.

Public Health

Heart failure is the leading cause of death amongst men and women which is why it is often the primary cause of concern amongst public health protagonists. Given this fact, American Heart Association feels that the U.S. Government does not take as much interest in the subject as it should. In fact it should keep track of the national rates of heart disease and stroke as doing so would help to curtail the frequency of this disease.

American Heart Association publishes an annual Heart Disease and Stroke journal in which all the data collected by different sources, such as magazines and surveys is published. Although the AHA has been doing a wonderful job compiling this information, it falls far short of being a complete study. In addition to this, the AHA is a nongovernmental agency and as such has no authority to modify the data collected. But for the doctors, these are the only sources to be relied upon to advance treatment protocols and hence, improvements in the field are slow.

While the Public Health Department keeps a record of other illnesses, this is not true of heart diseases. Although they are capable of supervising the method and scope of data collection and then evaluating and acting upon these results by implementing changes, they currently have no control. Thus the onus is on this department to ensure that everyone in the medical field has access to all the information pertaining to the heart and they can accomplish this by keeping track of heart patients.

People harbor the notion that the doctors that they rely on are fully informed on heart related disorders. On the contrary, owing to the lack of structure to any data collection method, there is severe shortage of information with only members of AHA making significant contributions. Even then the data that is collected by surveys requires modification to be of proper use to physicians in their capacity for treating heart patients. It is the responsibility of the Public Health Department to obtain this information from the primary physicians and some of systems that could be implemented to achieve this goal are -

Firstly, physicians should report heart disease and stroke whenever possible and also maintain laboratory reports on connected problems like unnaturally high blood sugar and cholesterol levels. This alone would make the information shared between doctors, and their patients, more available and comprehensive.

Secondly, the existing questions on risk factors for strokes, heart disease and other vascular diseases in the National surveys should be expanded to include factors like physical inactivity, smoking, obesity and unhealthy diet, to name a few.

Thirdly, the Public Health Department should review existing surveys and standardize the data collected in them to prevent duplication of information.

The Public Health Department is in service to everyone and the heart should be their main concern. Hence, starting to track patients with heart problems and maintaining records for the safety and well-being of all should be one of its first duties.

Medications

Maintaining a healthy heart depends heavily on using medications correctly, and understanding how the heart is affected by appropriate medication. There are different problems that affect the heart and each has separate treatment. So if a patient suffers from more than one problem, for example high blood pressure as well as cholesterol, then he would have to take separate medication for both.

There are a few basic groups of medications which are manufactured by pharmaceutical companies, who then attach their own names to them. For example Beta-Blockers, such as the medicine named Plavix, counteracts the hormone called noradrenalin. This, in turn, reduces the heart rate and the output of blood and hence is not suitable for people with severe heart failure. Patients who have high cholesterol take a drug called Lipitor, while those susceptible to strokes would take Nadolol. Another highly recommended medication is Bayer Aspirin 81mg, which is available over the counter and need not be prescribed. It is known to stop or prevent heart attacks. If in doubt about what basic group the medication falls into, asking the pharmacist is the best option.

A few other basic groups of medications that could be prescribed, depending on the specific heart condition are digitalis medicines, diuretics, Angiotensin Converting Enzyme (ACE) inhibitors and Angiotensin II Receptor Blockers (ARBS) and nitrate or hydralazine. Digitalis medicines improve circulation by increasing the force of the heart's contractions. Diuretics are prescribed to patients whose bodies retain fluid. ACE inhibitors were originally developed to treat high blood pressure by reducing the pressure in the blood vessels. This decreases the strain on the heart while it is trying to pump blood through the vessels, improves chances of survival for heart failure patients and slows or stops the loss of heart pumping activity. Similarly, the ARBS may also improve survival for heart failure patients and decrease or eliminate the loss of heart pumping activity. Where ACE inhibitors or ARBS cannot be taken, nitrate or hydralazine is prescribed instead for improving blood flow by causing the blood vessels to relax.

Taking medications correctly is imperative if a healthy heart is to be enjoyed. In the case of a 55-year-old man, the mismanagement proved fatal. Not wanting to take his medication with him on short weekend trips, this man would take all the medication prescribed for the weekend on the Friday afternoon preceding his trip. The first time he did so, he proclaimed that the room went round and he felt dizzy for a while. However, this did not alarm him sufficiently to begin taking it as advised and to his misfortune he did not make it the next time when he did this. It is vital that medications be taken only by doctors' prescription and exactly as per the manner of prescription. Not doing so could prove to be fatal for the patient because the heart is one of the most vital organs in our body and we need to take care of it if we want to survive.

What is the American Medical Association?

The American Medical Association (AMA) is a collaboration of doctors whose goal it is to further medical education and advance the medical care for all persons. It was founded at the University of Pennsylvania in 1847 and since then most of the issues pertaining to medicine and medical research have come under its purview.

Publication of the Journal of the American Medical Association (JAMA) is possibly the most commonly recognized achievement of the AMA. It is a peer reviewed scientific journal which is published forty eight times during the year and is the most widely circulated journal publication in the world. Being an encyclopedia on all health related fields, including public health and advancement in underprivileged countries, it maintains a high level of excellence through strict quality guidelines for submitted articles. It is invaluable for continuing education in all fields of medicine and is available free of charge to physicians in underdeveloped areas.

Another valuable tool, for clinicians and patients alike, is the website that has been established, www.ama-assn.org, where members of the AMA can be updated on current affairs. Throughout history this association has taken an active role in supporting or opposing medical legislation, such as the current Medicare controversy.

All health care professionals are required to complete a minimum number of credits per year for continuing education. The website lists opportunities such as these, as well as information concerning the HIPAA, an acronym for Health Insurance Portability and Accountability Act. This act dictates how third party claims should be submitted, particularly to insurance companies without violating the patient's privacy and leakage of personal medical information while still providing the patient with the care they need. This is a delicate balance to maintain.

Medical students can find valuable assistance on the website. Many are aided in enrolling in, and completing, medical school. They can also find a wide listing of possible medical careers. Financial aid, grants and scholarships are also available through the AMA as also financial advice for funding not obtained through the organization. In addition to this, students can seek help in selecting a medical school and are informed how to become licensed in their state of residency after completing their studies.

At the AMA's website, there is a button for non-physicians named DoctorFinder. By clicking on this patients can access the list of all doctors appropriately qualified to practice medicine in their chosen community who are registered with the AMA. Since they are also compliant with the standard of ethics established by the association, patients can search for a family physician, pediatrician or any other specialist as the need arises. Some doctors provide more information about themselves and their practice but it is mandatory for all listings to contain the name, address and phone number for the doctor, a detail that comes in handy in case of unfamiliar areas.

As an organization, the American Medical Association is devoted to bringing the best care and support to everyone, be it doctors, patients or students.

Epidemiology

The study of a disease or disorder is known as epidemiology. This process is conducted by an epidemiologist, whose task it is to measure the impact of a disease or disorder on the public and to interpret the rate/risk differences and the rate/risk ratios. Essentially, they define and carry out analysis, understand the results, as it pertains to the research and present these findings in a clear and concise manner. It is the role of the Public Health Department to conduct these studies to prevent diseases that are contagious in nature from spreading. Thus, employment of epidemiologists and the study of epidemiology via software packages like STATA, EPI-INFO and so on are of vital importance to the health and wellbeing of people.

To begin a study, the epidemiologist first needs to define and carry out the analysis. In order to do this a research problem needs to be established. Based on this, a study hypothesis can be formulated and the objectives of the study can be determined. Only then can the epidemiologist formulate the appropriate, and ethical, study design. This includes planning field procedures, determining the sample selection, setting the time frame for the study, and designing the questionnaires and record forms that will be used to compile the required data. These parameters are used to write up a detailed protocol, which, together with an estimated budget, is developed into a submission statement to be presented to a funding agency.

Once the data has been compiled, it needs to be interpreted. It is the task of the epidemiologist to decide which statistical methods would be best used to analyze simple data sets and then apply those methods by using appropriate computer software packages. The epidemiologist needs to understand the basic statistical measures and concepts used to analyze this data. The results are used to identify factors that indicate a disease is the result of infection. They are also needed to understand the factors that determine the distribution of communicable diseases in a spatial, temporal and social context. In addition to this, the epidemiologist has to understand the method behind measuring how the infection is transmitted and then is required to evaluate the efficacy of a vaccine. An outbreak investigation report can then be compiled using all of the information gathered.

The exceptional work done by epidemiologists is not always easy, but it is of vital importance in the prevention of major outbreaks of diseases. It is the duty of the Public Health Department to investigate diseases, and the American Heart Association feels that they have neglected the number one killer disease in America today – heart failure. The AHA has gathered as much information as possible through magazines, articles and a journal for doctors to refer themselves to. However, this is incomplete and inadequate to deal with the care and prevention of heart related diseases. The Public Health Department needs to provide an epidemiologist to study heart related diseases and devise a more thorough and comprehensive approach towards the prevention of heart failure.

Heart Failure

Cardiac conditions which damage or weaken the heart will ultimately lead to heart failure if ignored. A weakened heart would be unable to meet the day-to-day demands of the body and this would serve to stiffen its ventricles to the point that it would not fill properly between heartbeats. Over time, these ventricles would dilate and render the heart incapable of pumping and supplying blood to the entire body. Failure in pumping blood would force the fluid to back up and flood the circulatory system comprising of ankles, feet, legs and lungs. As a result, excess sodium and water would accumulate in the kidneys and such a build-up could trigger congestive heart failure. A left-sided heart failure causes fluids in the lungs build up to the point of causing congestion and this causes the right-side of the heart to fail too.

When the left side of the heart gets filled up with fluids, the right side of the heart feels the pressure of the lungs and this is what prevents it from functioning normally. The fluids would then travel down to the stomach and lower extremities, thus triggering a heart failure. A heart attack is usually followed by a heart failure, some of the underlying reasons being long-standing coronary artery disease or high blood pressure. However, there is another cause for heart failure namely a defective valve but this problem can be tackled by opting for heart valve replacement carried out by a cardiologist.

People are of the opinion that indulging in high-cholesterol and high-fat foods, obesity and smoking are common factors leading up to congestive heart failure. But then at times the heart can weaken with no apparent reason or explanation, this condition is called idiopathic dilated cardiomyopathy. Individuals suffering from this condition should contact a doctor immediately to prevent aggravation.

Heart failure could be attributed to simultaneous existence of several conditions which serve to weaken the heart over a period of time. Many a times, people suffer from such conditions and they are not even aware of it. Some of these conditions are:

- Coronary artery disease is the most common cause of heart failure. Atherosclerosis causes build-up of fat-rich deposits in the arteries termed as plaque which in turn leads to narrowing of blood vessel. Build-up of plaque is in turn responsible for weak or less vigorous pumping of the heart since it is deprived of oxygenated blood. Heart attack occurs when due to unstable plaque a blood clot is formed which immediately blocks the flow of blood to the heart muscle.

- Second most common reason for heart failure is hypertension or high blood pressure. In this condition, the heart has to work harder in order to pump the blood through the arteries and it is courtesy of overworking that causes its failure.

Maintaining a healthy weight and keeping physically fit through regular workouts are some of the suggestions made by a cardiologist to maintain a healthy heart and lifestyle.

Congestive Heart

If one has a congestive heart then paying adequate attention in form of frequent treatments is a must. Given the seriousness of this problem, even the government wishes to participate in finding effective cures and identifying preventive measures through investment of various resources.

A congestive heart would not be able to ensure sufficient circulation of blood in the human body, or the tissues to be precise and nor would it be able to pump out the venous blood coming into it. Therefore, cultivating an understanding of the functioning of this vital organ is imperative if heart failure is to be averted successfully.

While it is not possible to see through our chest to learn our heart's condition, this can be done by another method that entails maintaining alertness towards symptoms which are indicative of a problem. One of the signs of heart congestion that is commonly manifested is sudden shortness of breath when using the stairs or walking.

Those who feel very lethargic and tire frequently and easily, even though they have had a good rest may be suffering from this health condition. Thus, if you experience these symptoms along with other symptoms like swelling of abdomen, legs, ankles and feet, then it is time to visit a heart specialist. Congestive heart failure is also expressed through raspy breathing, constant coughing and wheezing. Manifestation of one or more of such symptoms should be sufficient reason to consult a physician immediately.

One might suddenly observe an increase in weight which continues despite being in a diet. This signifies a problem with your heart and is a very serious issue as it might be an indicator of a congestive heart. For these people, it is difficult to breathe, even when they might be supine. Congestive heart patients will cough and wheeze all the time and occasionally spit up red sputum too which is why timely treatment is imperative to prevent the problem from spinning out of control.

There are some serious symptoms associated with congestive heart failure, like palpitations of the heart and chest pain accompanied by fever. If this is happening to you then you should immediately rush to the emergency room as it marks the onset of congestive heart failure. Since it is necessary to nip the problem at the bud seeking help from a doctor is strongly recommended right at the initial stage. Generally the doctor would recommend that you visit a cardiologist, meaning heart specialist.

For making suggestions pertaining to the health of the heart, no-one would be better qualified than a cardiologist. In addition to a healthy lifestyle, he/she would also provide necessary treatment and draw up a good diet chart to enable the patient maintain a healthy heart. Just because you have congestive heart problems does not mean that congestive heart failure has to happen because as they say 'A stitch in time saves nine'.

Congestive Heart Failure Explained

It is but natural for patients to get absolutely petrified when they learn from their doctors that they have congestive heart failure because awareness pertaining to this condition is more or less negligible. For some odd reasons, people always think that congestive heart failure indicates the end of their lives and hence are warranted to react in this manner.

When the heart is weakened to the point of being unable to pump blood to the entire body in an effective manner the result is congestive heart failure. Now, since the heart muscles can get weak because of illness or overworking, heart failure can be categorized as a secondary disease which follows another cardiac condition. Cardiac arrhythmias, valvular diseases, myocarditis, cardiomyopathies and coronary artery disease are some of the culprits that cause congestive heart. Severe anemia or sepsis, renal failure and myocardial infarction also belong to the list but prognosis varies.

Our heart has two sides and because each differs from the other in terms of function, the impact on the body is also different. In case of failure of the left side, fluids would accumulate in the lungs, giving rise to difficulty in breathing and the kidneys would retain fluids too because of not receiving adequate blood supply. Likewise, if the right side of the heart fails then the venous system would suffer from accumulation of excess fluids, thereby causing a generalized edema in the patient which worsens with time.

One of the symptoms that all heart failure patients experience is dyspnea but of course its intensity differs from one patient to another. Some patients may have so many fluids accumulated in their body that even performing simple actions like getting up from the bed in the morning would require a mammoth effort. Others would remain perfectly normal until they start exerting their bodies through a variety of physical exercises. Because the tissues are deprived of adequate supply of oxygen from blood, therefore the patients tire very easily. A condition known as pitting edema also occurs in case of heart failure patients. In this condition a deep indentation or mark is left when pressure is applied to a particular spot on the patient's body.

In order to treat congestive heart failure, one must first treat the symptoms. Regular checking of vital signs and prescription of diuretics in order to expel accumulated excess fluids in the body needs to be carried out. Intake and output of fluids are monitored closely in hospitals and patients are usually asked to stay in an upright position in order to help the fluids move around the lungs and heart. Potassium supplements would also be given to the patients. The doctor would also monitor various levels pertaining to bicarbonate, chloride, potassium, sodium creatinine, sodium and BUN.

Factors like polycythemia, hypertension, anemia, malnutrition, obesity, use of drugs and alcohol abuse also causes congestive heart failure. Thus, such patients should make it a point to lead a very healthy lifestyle and follow a proper exercise plan to prevent excess stress on their lungs and heart. While there is no cure for congestive heart failure, it is certainly avoidable if one follows a healthy lifestyle, eats a balanced diet and exercises frequently.

Condition of Congestive Heart Failure Described

Our body can be defined as an awe-inspiring machine which works best when it is in tune with nature. All machines require replacement of parts from time to time, good care and measures to prevent breakdown and our heart is no exception to this rule. Functioning of a heart could be best described by drawing an analogy to a pump. When this experiences hindrance thanks to numerous core conditions, the outcome is congestive heart failure, a serious medical condition.

Since the human body grows weaker with time, the heart is capable of developing health problems like high blood pressure or coronary artery disease. Apart from causing congestive heart failure, these problems drain the heart of its strength and are irreversible and hence their incidence should be prevented by taking better care of one's body.

One way of increasing survival rate entails embarking on a course of medicines that would keep such health conditions under check. Such medications accomplish their objective by reducing and maintaining favorable cholesterol level, blood pressure and controlling any other factor that might impact the heart adversely. The fact that something as dreaded and deadly as congestive heart failure can now be prevented or averted is attributed to relentless advancements in the field of medicine.

Someone who is skilled enough to perform by-pass surgery a.k.a stents for opening up the blocked arteries and helping blood gush through the veins could only be a heart specialist, also known as cardiologist. Amongst the many possible solutions that one can adopt in order to stay healthy, simply seeking advice from the doctor as what would be best suited to the physiology is probably the best.

Implementing changes in one's lifestyle plays an instrumental role in preventing congestive heart failure. While this may not completely turn things around, it does make life easier to a degree. First things first, a healthy diet is a must followed by reduction in consumption of fats and salt because overindulgence could be regrettable. Improving one's quality of life also helps, and this can be done by learning to overcome occasional depression and stress. Obesity is also a nuisance as it is the root cause of many health problems like coronary artery disease and high sugar, cholesterol and blood pressure. For good health, it is important to keep weight under check.

For a lot of people, the task of managing stress is probably just short of impossible. Because of the busy and hectic lifestyle, one does not have the time, space and money to allow the heart to roll in the lap of luxury. Allowing the tension to build up in the heart is definitely a huge blunder because we need to give our heart a break from all the emotions it emotes - excitement, sadness, happiness and depression.

Prevention being better than cure is certainly applicable in case of congestive heart failure and prevention, in this case means to start afresh and make things turn around for best results.

Evidence Collaborating Diagnosis of Congestive Heart Failure

True though it may be that cardiac conditions are characterized with symptoms of difficult breathing and chest pain, congestive heart failure is an exception because it has very specific symptoms and lab results. Thus doctors can rely on very firm clues to make a definitive diagnosis of this condition.

A conclusive evidence for congestive heart failure would be laborious breathing, also known as dyspnea, followed by severe pitting edema. The latter is a condition wherein the body retains so much fluid that it can preserve an object's imprint that has been kept pressed for some time. Heart failure prevents the heart from efficiently pumping blood and thus, it causes retention of fluids and makes an individual bloat up like a balloon. Those having fluid retention bereft of imprints, meaning non-pitting edema are safe from heart failure, although they are liable to cough up frothy pink sputum.

Some of the problems experienced frequently by heart failure patients are malaise and a general feeling of weakness when they exert themselves physically. Such symptoms should not be ignored as they are caused by shortage of nourishment supplied by the blood to the tissues. If neglected for an extended duration these are capable of creating permanent damage to the organs. Another sure-shot symptom of heart failure is the lack of urination. Anuria, as it is sometimes called, happens because fluids cannot be excreted and remain accumulated in the tissues, hence causing the patient's mental status to suffer due to enhanced toxicity.

Blood samples and physical evidence are tested in laboratories by physicians for the purpose of confirming heart failure. A highly effective screening tool for detecting this condition would be a hormone known as BNP, Beta-natriuretic peptide, whose production increases when the fluid levels rise and the heart muscles fail. The level of BNP in case of a congestive heart failure is between 100-500 pg/mg and anything greater than this is conclusive. However, high BNP does not always translate into heart failure and could also indicate hypoxia, tumors, ventricular strain and renal failure.

To determine the extent of hypoxemia, arterial blood gasses need to be tested. Patients during the early or moderate stages of hypoxemia would suffer from elevated blood urea level, proteinuria or protein present in urine and a reduced erythrocyte sedimentation rate. Patients suffering from advanced cases of congestive heart failure would experience symptoms like increased bilirubin in the blood and decreased serum sodium levels.

In order to study the heart, radiology could come in handy. Fluid surrounding the heart and its enlargement can be detected by a chest x-ray and any structural abnormalities like mitral stenosis could be detected by performing an echocardiogram. This helps doctors in identifying the presence of heart failure particularly in case of valvular heart disease.

Doctors work like detectives when it comes to the task of diagnosing heart failure as they run evaluation tests, gather evidences and study them to reach a conclusion. Based on these findings, they provide the necessary treatment to the patient.

Emergence of New Therapies

One of the most fatal killers around the world today is heart disease and secondary to other cardiac diseases is a condition known as congestive heart failure. Given its high mortality rate, out of all people diagnosed with the disease at least half of the victims succumb within five years. There is a race to not only understand the disease and exact mechanisms but find a cure by researchers and scientists.

When the heart cells are rendered useless or die because of a heart attack or ischemia a person begins to experience congestive heart failure. No matter what the cause is the heart is unable to pump sufficient blood through the entire body. This results in formation of blood pools throughout the organs while fluid starts accumulating in and around the lungs. Since the body is no longer capable of discarding sodium through normal physiological methods, dyspnea, the classic symptom of congestive heart failure, sets in.

Possible treatment of the disease and repairing damaged heart cells are two areas that are targeted by clinical research. There is research going on right now for testing new medications that could possibly assist with vasodilation. Quest is also on for a calcium inhibitor that could help result in lower incidences of any cardiac arrhythmia seen when using medications available in the market today.

In case of patients suffering from heart failure stress has been found to be the main culprit. Application of naturopathy has helped towards strengthening of mind and there are clinical trials underway where techniques of relaxation and meditation are being used to combat stress faced by the heart. When the heart muscle is weak it is forced to work harder to pump the blood in spite of the stress slowing it down. A theory that when a body is capable of maintaining a lower level of stress it will cause the heart to relax is being tested and might work in favor of the patient.

Another recent development is that of clinical technology wherein scientists believe they have found the pair of altered genes that are responsible for making individuals more likely to suffer congestive heart failure. They are using their knowledge of current genes in combination with the benefits of therapy to try and reverse the symptoms. There are treatment programs already in place utilizing medications like alpha 2 agonists and beta blockers which tend to clamp down on this gene's activities.

The hitherto unexplored arena of stem cell usage, the body's own pluripotent progenitors, for assisting in the repair of damaged tissue in the heart is also being seriously considered. Clinical trials have shown when patients suffering from congestive heart failure were injected with their own stem cells the response was positive. It has been suggested that the cells either encourage other cells to come to the heart to help repair the cells or they actually help with the growth of any new vessels in the heart.

Scientists have been testing growing tissue that is healthy from the embryonic stem cells by transplanting them. There is a lot of controversy though because in order to get embryonic stem cells the embryo has to be destroyed. Unfortunately scientists have come to the conclusion that stem cells from adults do not provide enough numbers of the new cells for meeting the needs of heart failure patients.

Since the body is not capable of reproducing dead tissue cells of the heart, patients run the risk of being diagnosed with heart failure. Researchers have not given up hope that one day they will find a cure as modern advancements become better.

In U.S. Mortality Rate Is Lower By 28% in Top Hospitals

In a study conducted on hospitals in terms of their mortality rates by the American Heart Association, it was revealed that in the entire nation the top hospitals boasted of a mortality rate that was lower by 28%. On the 29th of January 2007 an independent health care ratings company called Health Grades released this information. It also observed that a patient undergoing surgery at one of the top rated hospitals was less susceptible to procedural complications.

There were 26 procedures along with diagnosis that Health Grades analyzed for mortality and death rates. These included heart attack, angioplasty, bypass surgery, and stroke, at a total of 5,122 hospitals considered nonfederal. The death rate average was found to be reduced by 11.7% and complications rates from post-surgery were less by 3.4% in the top hospitals. As per the author, if all hospitals in the U.S. offered the same top quality care as the crème de la crème then as many as 158,264 lives would not have been lost and there would have been 12,409 less major complications. Health Grades was sad to report a huge hiatus existing between the top hospitals and other hospitals across the U.S.

If hospitals met the minimum parameters like patient volume, ratings in quality, and range of services offered then they would be eligible to feature on Health Grades list. As per this, 229 hospitals located throughout the nation constituting the top five percent emerged as ones that provide uncompromising care to heart patients. At the top of the list for providing cardiovascular care was Christ Hospital, Cincinnati, Ohio and it is affiliated with other hospitals in that area which also rank in the top 100 of the five percent.

Robert Wood Johnson's University Hospital located in the state of New Jersey is a noteworthy name in this category because when it comes to patient safety and clinical quality this hospital remains unparalleled. Since it is the top teaching hospital of the University of Medicine in the state, it is in an intimidating position.

Another reputed name is that of Dayton Heart Hospital when it comes to dealing with heart problems and fighting related circumstances as a part of patient care. There is no other disease that kills more each year than heart disease which is why the quest is on for seeking new and better ways for healing patients. As a society the impact of heart disease is being reduced because of collective efforts of all sections of the community.

A heart wing has been renovated in Grand Rapids, Michigan at Spectrum Hospital and it has now become a leading center for transplants and open heart surgeries. The staff here understands the levels of stress as also the needs of patients and so they go out of their way to help in any way possible. Patient care continues even after the patient is discharged from the hospital in form of provision of home nurses who visit the patient every day to ensure they are not having any problems. When the patient is ready for therapy, application of therapy techniques by professionals in the therapy wing is carried out and a diet plan is chalked out by the dietician. All this care ensures the patient will have exemplary care aimed towards achieving complete recovery.

A Healthy Heart Keeps Congestive Heart Failure Away

Congestive heart failure patients are increasing in number so there was a meeting held at American College of Cardiology for discussing some controversial findings and brainstorming about how to provide better treatment. Since everyone is different the treatments will also be varied, meaning one treatment for patient A may not work for patient B. From the patient's perspective, confusion reigns supreme regarding whether they are getting the proper treatment for the heart condition they were diagnosed with.

When a study was conducted comparing drug therapy with angioplasty the results turned out to be the same over 2,300 patients. It did not matter if the patients were treated only with medication or if they were on medication alongside stinting and angioplasty because the outcome was the same in case of deaths, heart attacks, strokes or even hospitalization.

People know their bodies and hence are cognizant with the requisite dosage of diet and exercise – this is an assumption that the physician rely on. The medical field has to treat patients based on their individual requirement of any medical procedures. All patients should be told what their care is going to be as also how they can go about preventing congestive heart failure. Every patient needs to have a plan in place for taking action and having a healthy lifestyle like eating right and getting plenty of exercise.

It is within the patient's right to decide the type of treatment they would like to receive as per their body types. When experiencing any sort of symptoms write them down on paper and discuss with a doctor. This would help the doctor to diagnose what is wrong and the treatment that should be given. If a patient is ever in doubt about the treatment plan chalked out by doctor then getting a second opinion is in order. In case there are symptoms of congestive heart failure or if the doctor says it is likely to happen in the near future then take action and start a program.

If a person is overweight then they should look into an appropriate diet program that fits into his physical needs so that the weight can not just be shed but stay off too. This does not mean joining a weight loss program and investing a lot of money into special foods. Surf the Internet and take a look at the free diets. Having identified a plan, make an appointment with the doctor to check suitability. Exercising will also need to come in with the diet to help with the weight loss and relieve stress. Keep journals of everything including vitals, a weekly weight chart, and anything else that may seem important because after all it is your heart and your life that is at stake.

Congestive Heart Failure Can Be Combated With Doctors Skills

Many patients do not recognize the symptoms of congestive heart failure because the onset is not only slow but covert as well. As the condition worsens, patients will suffer from edema and dyspnea. When they seek treatment, they will be informed by the doctor that their heart is not functioning as it should.

Over time the heart tissue cells are destroyed or rendered nonfunctional due to a cardiac issue which is different from usual causes of heart failure like ischemic or coronary. It means that the patient's heart is not pumping adequate blood to the rest of their body and instead it is pooling along the way. As a result, organs become starved for oxygen and malfunction, meaning instead of fluids being excreted through the body they are now retained. Everyone knows when brain cells die they cannot be replaced - it is exactly the same with the heart cells too. Mortality rate for congestive heart failure is high and once the diagnosis is made more than half the victims actually succumb to the disease within the next five years. Advancements in medicine have enabled researchers discover ways in which the patient could be helped and there are even cases where the doctor is able to make a prognosis in favor of the patient.

Unfortunately the patient is usually not even aware of the presence of the disease until he lands up in the Emergency Wing complaining of laborious breathing and incessant chest pain. While in the hospital he will be stabilized by the doctors who would put him on a supply of supplemental oxygen and then follow it up with commencement of medicinal treatment to enable him to go home.

Congestive heart failure damage is being combated with a number of methods administered by doctors thanks to modern science. After the oxygen levels have been restored the physician will be able to administer a diuretic. This serves to stimulate the patient's renal system so the fluid can be pulled out of circulation and relieve the lungs, heart and other body organs from the stress of handling edema. Supplemental potassium is also simultaneously injected because the renal system removes potassium along with any excess fluid, thus rendering the threat of hypokalemia very real.

Angiotensin II is known for aggravating congestive heart failure so the medicine field has decided to focus on its characteristics as also method of production. Our body produces Angiotensin II which in addition to raising the blood pressure also causes constriction of blood vessels, thus hindering the heart's ability to pump the blood to the various body parts. In order to stop the body from producing angiotensin II an inhibitor called ACE is administered. If a patient's body does not respond to this then an angiotensin receptor blocker like nitroglycerin is used.

Congestive heart failure research is ongoing and within the science community there is a lot of debate raging about the use of stem cells, particularly the embryonic variety, being used as a treatment for heart failure. There have been patients who were diagnosed with heart failure and when injected with their own stem cells, experienced improvement. However, scientists are not sure if the stem cells are aiding the body in growing new vessels or are acting like a lighthouse sending warning signals so that other cells are drawn to the site of damage. No matter what the case might be using stem cells has presented doctors with an opportunity wherein they could try restoring functions of the heart for the hapless victims.

With so many new treatment options courtesy of modern science, patients of congestive heart failure can look forward to the future anew. Researchers are constantly pushing for new frontiers and soon enough there will be a day when medicine will be able to unravel the riddle of successfully treating heart failure.

Saving the Heart Medically

Congestive heart failure does not have a cure but you can take a number of steps towards prolonging your life while shielding your heart from more deterioration. Improvement in quality of life will come from lifestyle changes and drug therapy with the former including no-smoking, loss of excess weight, consumption of less alcohol and eating healthy by eliminating salty and foods with saturated fat content. Pair these changes with exercising a few times a week and now you are on your way for preventing heart failure. If diagnosed with the disease never try and prescribe medications for treatment on your own and instead visit a physician and let them give you the proper medical treatment.

Just like other organs in your body, there are different ways in which the heart can malfunction. This is where a cardiologist comes in and one of the ways that he can tackle the problem is by prescribing a beta blocker. This medicine functions by counteracting with the hormone noradrenalin so the blood output is increased while reducing your heart rate. But if you have suffered severe heart failure then this medication is not for you.

There are times when fluid buildup or even high blood pressure is observed in patients and when this happens the doctor might prescribe a diuretic. Despite the compensation that it provides, the user should be wary of possible side effects like potassium loss, cramping of muscles, pains in the joints, and even weakness. If you experience any of these symptoms while using a diuretic, let your doctor know immediately.

Apart from these, the medical field can aid in preventing heart failure through other treatments that are equally effective. The medical field knows how extreme congestive heart failure can be that is why they have been experimenting with mechanical pumps which attach to the heart and heart transplants. There are now a few medical centers in the U.S. that are offering an experimental procedure known as cardiomyoplasty. It involves going into the back and detaching an end of the muscle and wrapping it carefully around the heart, and suturing it in place. An electric stimulator is implanted to cause the muscle in the back to contract so blood can be pumped from the heart.

There is another option known as mitral valve repair which will help correct any leaky valves that have resulted from cardiomyopathy. A flexible annuloplasty ring is surgically inserted at the opening of the mitral valve thus serving not only to improve lives but extend them as well for victims of congestive heart failure.

Thanks to the medical field and the strides in medicine and surgical procedures people can now look forward to improving their quality of life. Healthy diets and exercises, according to experiments conducted by the medical field, are equally contributory and hence can be adopted by anyone who truly cares for their heart.

Understanding the Impact and Living with It

The knowledge of living with heart failure is a frightening thought for anyone suffering from it, but there is a chance for you to be able to lead a normal life by planning and discussing an effective treatment regime with your cardiologist. By doing so, instead of the diagnosis being the beginning of an end it could well be the gateway leading to a healthier and happier lifestyle.

When your heart does not pump blood properly throughout the body heart failure occurs. The blood pools deprive organs of oxygen and nutrients and the fluid retention that takes place due to excess sodium not been excreted through urine. This leads to dyspnea and stress in organs. A patient may die if left untreated due to death of cells in organs resulting in organ failure.

Medications are available and are prescribed by your physician which aid in proper flow of blood, taking the pressure off the heart, thinning the blood, reducing clot formation in the veins, helping you to prolong life. Apart from medication alteration of life style also has an impact on your disease progression.

Both rest and exercise in sensible doses is important for your heart. Similar to resting a leg after injury, resting the heart enables it to pump blood efficiently throughout the body. The exercise regime has to be considered carefully with your physician and established according to what works best for you. Exercise does not need to be extensive physical workouts and a walk every day for half an hour is sufficient.

Working out a diet plan with your physician is as essential as working out an exercise regime. A diet low in sodium aids in reducing the retention of fluid. If a diuretic is prescribed a supplement of daily potassium will also be prescribed as diuretics change the levels of potassium in the body. Change in levels of potassium leads to hypokalemia, resulting in paralysis, muscle weakness and fatal cardiac arrhythmia and hence restoration of this element within the body is imperative.

It is essential that once diagnosed with heart failure, you should stop smoking with immediate affect. Nicotine causes an increase in heart rate and blood pressure, and can cause reduction in levels of oxygen in the blood, thus exerting your heart.

Contacting flu or pneumonia caused by the pneumococcal bacteria is detrimental when diagnosed with heart failure. Staying away from crowded areas and people known to be sick usually works. Apart from this, receiving the annual flu vaccine and pneumococcal vaccination is deemed helpful when you are diagnosed with heart failure. Contacting pneumonia is as problematic as smoking as it causes the similar effects, meaning it reduces the levels of oxygen in the blood exerting the heart and adding to the stress.

Also wearing loose fitting clothes is useful for patients living with heart failure. When clothes are tight it can restrict blood flow to the extremities and aid in the clotting of blood. Apart from this if your body has to exert itself in order to maintain its temperature the heart will again be under stress as it will be forced to work harder. Therefore wearing appropriate clothing according to the changing weather patterns relieves the stress on the heart to a great extent.

Discussion about sexual relationships with a physician is also useful for a person diagnosed with heart failure particularly if your condition is severe. It may be a good idea to refrain from sex or from intense sexual practices. However if your condition is not severe, a normal sexual relationship can be continued if it is conducted in an environment that does not cause unwanted stress.

The fact that heart failure will adversely affect a person's life style is inevitable but it is up to you to decide its degree of influence. If each of the above steps is followed closely it will aid in prolonging life and help you to enjoy life to the fullest.

Finding Current Research

For a common man not associated with the field of medicine finding information pertaining to a particular disease and treatment options available is a tedious process. Research data provides information, with numerous sources but how valuable and useful are they to a common man is a question that needs to be answered. Physicians attend conferences and research forums to keep up with field which is constantly changing, but the commoner is left to browse through a vast amount of information and sources and derive his own conclusions. Therefore the best method is to read several journals and articles thoroughly before reaching a conclusion.

A journal dedicated exclusively to a certain topic is rather difficult to find. If therefore a person requires finding information on congestive heart failure he or she would have to read a countless number of journals published. These are found both as hard copies and soft copies online. A patient can subscribe to a particular journal he or she is interested in if the information required is present in it. This enables them to find new information as it is released. Journals can be found in libraries and also online. Online subscriptions allow a part of published work to be accessed without a subscription, where as several periodicals can be acquired through libraries with subscriptions. It is always advantageous to read more than one journal as information on a particular topic can be found in multiple sources rather than in one.

Revolutionary research is found in scientific journals. This aids the common man to get in touch with the latest progress in all fields of science including medicine. It takes a person to research laboratories across the globe, providing insight to what the future holds for the world. For example when information on stem cell research was first published it proved to be controversial but now it is considered as one of the best methods for providing a cure for patients with heart failure.

One thing to keep in mind when reading articles is that the source it is from is in fact reliable. Hypothesis and factual information are both present in journal articles and the difference between them needs to be determined. For a patient for whom science is foreign, it is best to speak to his or her physician and with the help of the physician read journals which contain accurate and precisely reviewed articles, which can provide the patient with proper information. Reading journals that publish hypothetical information can be detrimental to a patient with a limited knowledge in medical research.

For a layman to understand a scientific journal with its infinite information it is best to have a physician to consult and always be armed with a medical dictionary, as medical jargon is difficult to understand. It is also worthwhile to keep in mind that these articles are written by health professionals with specifically health professionals in mind. Therefore, the physician and medical dictionary are very useful.

Importance of Peer Review in Publication of Medical Research

It is essential to read articles in scientific journals that are peer reviewed when searching for latest research carried out in the medical field. Peer reviewed journals provide the reader with precise and current data.

Publishers of magazines such as Cosmo, Time, Good Housekeeping and many other periodicals we are familiar with do not allow for peer review. It is the editor who makes a decision if an article is suitable to publish or not. However an editor can always make a mistake in facts, as it is not humanly possible for a person to know everything. Personal opinions, baseless statements, prejudiced investigations, meaningless research data are printed in articles. If a reader is searching for such articles it is excellent reading material, but for someone in a quest for facts it is a different matter altogether. This problem is then addressed and rectified as much as possible when journals are peer reviewed.

Peer reviewing or refereeing (as known to scientists) is a straight forward process. Initially all research articles to be published are submitted to the editor of the specific journal. Thereafter copies of each article in a specific subject area are handed over to two or three professionals specialized in that subject area. For example articles pertaining to congestive heart failure will be submitted to several cardiologists. These professionals who are the "peers" of the authors, then assess the article for precision or accuracy, quality and significance to the journal the author desires it to be published in. They hand over their assessment to the editor of the journal. By this it is decided if the article is worth publishing in a particular journal. As we can see a great deal of expertise goes into deciding the publication of each article.

Reviewers in the past had been anonymous to authors as well as to the general public, thus preventing authors from challenging his or her reviews. However, there are instances where editors have allowed authors to refute a criticism of their work made by a reviewer, if in case the article in question has received mixed reviews. At present the system is undergoing a gradual change and open peer review systems are been utilized, where reviewer's names are published and can be held answerable for their comments. The Journal of Interactive Media in Education for example was among the first to use the open peer review system.

Journals which have been subjected to peer reviewing are more dignified, use technical language extensively and have citations of all sources and therefore can be distinguished easily from others. These are directed more towards professionals in the field and are focused on scientific research than general topics. There are sources now available across the country for scholars to know for certain if journal publications have undergone peer review or not.

Treating Congestive Heart Failure

The failure of the heart to pump blood to satisfy the needs of the body is known as congestive heart failure. This has devastating effects on the body. Physicians try treating symptoms and strive to give patients the best cure, but no method for complete cure currently exists.

When the heart is unable to pump blood properly throughout the body, the nutrients and oxygen are not distributed. The excess fluid is not excreted into the urine, instead, the starts pooling. This triggers fluid retention resulting in edema. Fluid building up in the veins results in localized edema, with swelling of the extremities, whereas fluid building up in the organs results in systemic edema, resulting in swelling of the organs. The fluid accumulation puts an excessive amount of stress on the heart and as fluid accumulates in the pleural cavity it results in dyspnea or difficulty in breathing, which is symptomatic of heart failure. The swelling, lack of oxygen and nutrients to the organs lead to permanent damage to the organs. This if left untreated provides a poor outcome for the patient.

Treatment is administered in several stages. In the first stage, treatment consists of the administration of extra oxygen, in order to normalize oxygen levels in the tissues. Once oxygen is administered, a pulse oximeter is used to reveal if the blood oxygen levels are acceptable. Once this is done the next treatment targets the fluid buildup in the body. Diuretics are administered to assist the excess fluid out of the body through the urinary tract. When treating with diuretics the body excretes potassium in the urine, which leads to long term hypokalemia resulting in muscle weakness and paralysis as well as an increased risk of cardiac arrhythmia. Therefore supplemental potassium has to be administered along with diuretics. Nitrates are then administered to cause the vessels to dilate, which allows the blood to flow more freely, relieving heart of its load.

ACE (angiotensin-converting-enzyme) inhibitors which prevent the body from creating angiotensin together with diuretics are given to patients on discharge. Angiotensin raises blood pressure and causes blood vessels to constrict. An angiotensis II receptor blocker is also administered if production of angiotensin continues. If patients have responded poorly to treatment with ACE inhibitors in the past then vasodilators other than ACE inhibitors, such as nitroglycerin are administered.

To strengthen the force of the heart's contraction and helping to push the blood through the body, drugs such as Digitalis or Digoxin are prescribed. To prevent the heart from beating rapidly, trying to compensate for the poor movement of the blood and placing more stress on the already weakened heart, the patient may be given a beta blocker. Coumadin and heparin, the commonly prescribed blood thinners may be included to prevent clot formation in the blood vessels. However patients taking these medications should undergo coagulation testing regularly as there is an increased risk of bleeding.

Apart from long term medication patients with heart failure should strive to change their life style as well. Patients should avoid smoking, as nicotine from cigarettes increases the heart rate, blood pressure and clotting in the blood vessels. Patients should also be vaccinated against flu with the annual influenza vaccine and with the pneumococcal vaccine, which will protect them from the pneumococcal bacteria which causes over eighty percent (80%) of bacterial pneumonia. Also to be considered is the clothing which should be loose fitting to aid in blood flowing into the extremities and preventing clots. Body should always be at an appropriate temperature during extreme warm or cold temperatures.

A complete cure for congestive heart failure is still under research. It is of vital importance therefore for patients to follow the treatment regime prescribed by their physician. If patients adhere to all advice and treatment regimes, there is a dramatic improvement of life in a patient suffering from congestive heart failure.

Ways Patients Can Take Advantage of Translational Research

The outcome of a particular treatment performed on a laboratory test animal may or may not be the same when performed on a human test subject. For the results of such research to be effective, findings have to be taken to the clinic and this forms the essence of translational research. After all, the adage – every action has an equal and opposite reaction, may not stand fully validated in science since the reaction is subject to variation.

In the first stage of translational research, controlled clinical treatment trials are performed on a voluntary group of test subjects. If these tests meet the acceptable range of success, the treatment is then taken to research hospitals such as the St. Jude's Children's Research Hospital in Boston, USA. Here patients are subjected to the new method of treatment, with the understanding that it is still in an experimental stage. However for many, these treatments represent a ray of hope that was hitherto completely out of reach for them.

One area in which translational research can be applied is congestive heart failure (CHF). At the moment this disease is believed to be deadly because the cells of the heart muscle are destroyed and the heart no longer can pump blood adequately throughout the body. With no replacement for the destroyed cells, it is impossible for the heart to regain its full function. Considering the fact that over fifty percent (50%) of patients die within five years after being diagnosed with this problem, the current mortality rate of CHF is high. There are many treatment options currently under consideration like Montefiore Medical Centre in New York is performing clinical trials using a drug known as "Lovosimendan" which is a calcium sensitizer that does not trigger cardiac arrhythmia. Researchers are also studying the possibility of using stem cells to re-grow cardiac tissues.

The patient, if willing to take advantage of the ongoing clinical trials by being a test subject, must discuss the matter with his or her physician. On finding the so-called patient a good potential candidate, the physician may then refer him to the research facility or suggest the patient's name for the clinical trial. If a patient lives in an area already having a hospital carrying out research, there is an opportunity for him or her to benefit from the hospitals policy on translational research.

What has to be understood is that translational research is still in its 'research' phase with medical researchers still grasping its mode of treatment and its effect on the human body. The possibility of the treatment being unsuccessful with hazardous side effects unknown to medical world is always present. But, for patients who have lost "hope", even with its negative side effects, translational research provides the last straw that the trials would work and they will be cured. It also provides future patients who will be diagnosed with similar diseases with faith in the treatment method, thanks to the patients who volunteer to be test subjects in translational research.

How Can Stem Cells Be Used to Treat Congestive Heart Failure?

Congestive heart failure occurs when the heart cells are destroyed or not functioning properly, thus making it difficult for the heart to circulate blood through the body. In some cases, patients can receive mechanical aids or heart transplants, but this is not always possible. The damage that is done to the body is immense and, in spite of the best efforts of researchers and physicians, the result is frequently lasting organ damage and, ultimately, death. Researchers are confident that stem cells may be the answer to this lethal problem.

A lot of medical journals have focused their attention on the possibilities of using stem cells. In adults, stem cells are mainly produced in the bone marrow. If this is not possible due to a crisis, such as in the case of leukemia, other organs which contain stem cells during the development of a fetus, e.g. the spleen, take over from the bone marrow. In this way, the body can keep the correct balance, replacing cells as they die. Red blood cells, only in the circulatory system for about four months, start off as rubriblasts produced by the hematopoietic stem cells found within the bone marrow. This is an adult form of stem cell.

Researchers are also focusing on embryonic stem cells because they are not limited to what cell they can develop into and they can provide many cells that replenish themselves. These pluripotent cells are found in blastocysts, four to five day old human embryos, which divide and increase to eventually develop into the body and internal organs of the fetus. Unfortunately, the harvesting of these embryonic stem cells usually results in the destruction of the embryo, which makes their use highly controversial.

Recently, a number of techniques have been discussed in research journals relating to the use of stem cells to treat congestive heart failure. In one group of patients, a number of years ago, there were no other treatment options and so they agreed to participate in a stem cell test. Autologous stem cells from the marrow were removed and injected through the chest wall and into the damaged portion of the heart. They showed a notable improvement and the assumption is that the stem cells were responsible. Research scientists believe that the stem cells have either grown new vessels to replace the unhealthy ones, or they have attracted other cells to repair the damage.

Along another avenue of research, stem cells could be used to grow new heart tissue in a laboratory. Stem cells are not stimulated to differentiate produce pluripotent daughter cells in a laboratory. The tissue that forms can easily adapt to suit the environment it is placed in. In this way, heart tissue can be grown and transplanted into a patient who suffers from heart failure and the damaged, dead tissue can be replaced with living tissue. Since hearts are not very easy to procure for transplants, and the waiting lists extend over years, this procedure would give a patient a better functioning heart and hopefully a better opportunity to survive.

At least half of the patients diagnosed with congestive heart failure will die before five years. The other half will be severely affected by their heart failure for the rest of their lives. Research into stem cells offers a chance of hope for heart failure patients, that perhaps they can win this battle.

How Can Continuing Medical Education Credits Be Obtained?

The field of medicine is an immense subject, perpetually changing and growing. It is not possible for a physician to learn everything there is to know, even after spending numerous years studying towards their MD. Continued medical education (CME) is vital for physicians to remain apprised of the latest developments, discoveries, and treatments in their particular field

Forty years ago, or even twenty years ago, the medicine practiced was very different and what worked then may not be the best treatment available now. Physicians are allocated a certain number of continuing education credits per year which need to be completed. Although they can complete more credits if they so wish, not completing them would put their patients' lives in danger, because they would be unaware of the treatments found to be harmful or not as effective as latest introductions.

Fortunately, there are more convenient ways to earn these credits than returning to school. If the physician wanted to spare time and work for investing in school then they certainly would, but most have very little time left after caring for their patients. There are many symposiums, conferences, workshops and medical conventions all over the country which address many subjects. Often they are held over a weekend and extend over two or more days. Physicians from anywhere in the nation can go to whichever location suits them best. The latest surgical technique used in the treatment of collapsed heart valves, using stem cells in the treatment of congestive heart failure, and other developments, which are too new to be found in a medical school, are taught here.

Although doctors in rural areas may find it difficult to attend, there are still options available for them to complete their continuing medical education credits. Very often they are the only doctor their patients have and, as such, are on call twenty four hours per day. They treat patients from birth to death and everything in between - treating toothaches and heart attacks alike and taking their own rounds in the hospital. There is no time for them to leave their patients and practice for a weekend. Fortunately, the internet is a vast new resource in the field of continuing education. The American Medical Association (AMA), the American Association for Continuing Medical Education (AACME), and other organizations, offer options for completing continuing medical education credits online. Online, physicians can complete coursework, view conferences and even sit at symposiums and lectures using the teleweb.

All these CME resources are either offered for free or they can charge per credit hour at a low rate. It depends on the individual situation. Still, this is less expensive and time consuming than it would be to return to college or university, and more up to date.

Continuing medical education provides physicians with the opportunity to remain informed of the best and most innovative options for caring for patients in their field. This benefits the patients as well as the physicians. The learning never stops, particularly in the medical field.

Enjoy the Highest Quality of Life Possible With CHF

Congestive heart failure arises if the cells of the heart have difficulty contracting as they should, and so they are less able to circulate blood through the body. Dyspnea, is a shortness of breath that is typical of heart failure, is caused by the resultant edema found in the body, especially in and around the lungs. Getting a diagnosis such as this, impacts upon every aspect of life and many changes in lifestyle may be required. Foregoing much loved activities, changing eating patterns and possibly even discarding clothing may make a patient resent the sacrifices they have had to make for their health. There are a number of things patients suffering with heart failure can do to enjoy the life they are saving.

The edema can be controlled by prescription diuretics and a low sodium diet. This allows the fluid excesses to leave via the renal system and this makes breathing more manageable. Although daily exercise is essential, it is possible that patients will need to modify activities they have enjoyed thus far, if they put too much strain on the heart. Any exercise plan should be approved by the physician to ensure that it is not too vigorous. Still, as long as caution is maintained, physical activity can be varied and adaptable.

Another essential component of living with congestive heart failure is rest. The body needs time, scheduled each day, to regain its strength. This may include reading, watching television, napping or meditating. Meditation is being focused on to treat heart failure patients. It reduces the heart rate, normalizes the blood pressure, reduces the amount of adrenalin produced, and helps the muscles to use oxygen more efficiently. All these factors help to decrease the strain on the heart.

Smoking is especially harmful for patients with heart failure. Nicotine increases the blood pressure and heart rate while preventing oxygen from reaching the muscles and impeding circulation by making the blood thicken and adhere to the blood vessels. This forces the heart to work harder and places more strain on the weakened organ.

Another thing to be avoided as much as possible is flu and pneumonia. Both these illnesses reduce the oxygen in the blood, forcing the heart to beat harder in compensation. Avoiding areas with large crowds during cold and flu season will help, as will vaccines. At least one dose of pneumococcal vaccine protects against the pneumococcal bacteria, which commonly causes bacterial pneumonia. An annual influenza vaccination will help ward off the flu.

Even clothing can affect a patient's health. Patients suffering from congestive heart failure should wear loose clothing and dress appropriately for the weather. Restrictive clothing and stockings increase the risk of blood clots and blockages in the blood flow to the limbs. Excessive temperatures also need to be avoided. The harder the body needs to work to regulate its temperature, the more strain is exerted on the heart.

Above all else, patients suffering from heart failure need to enjoy their life. It is a well-known fact that stress has a negative effect on the heart. Patients with a positive mental attitude, and who avoid stress, create a healthier environment for their hearts. A happy, stress free existence is therefore emotionally and physically beneficial.

Continuing Medical Education for Cardiac Professionals

Change is inevitable. This is especially true of the medical field. Almost every day new information, different diseases, and diverse symptoms in each patient are discovered by researchers. So how do health care professionals synchronize their knowledge with the changes? One way is through continuing education.

Although a cardiologist takes upward of twelve years to earn his degree, each year new treatments and surgeries are developed, resources and technology are enhanced, new opportunities arise and more knowledge is added to the field. Treatments can be ruled ineffective or even unsafe for patients, and are replaced by new modes. So after undergrad school, medical school, residency, and finally coursework and residency for specialization, the cardiologist will still not know everything, and never will. They will always need to keep learning. But since we need our physicians to treat us, not spend all their time sitting in classrooms and lecture halls, this is where the continuing education comes in.

There are a predetermined number of continuing education credits that need to be completed by physicians, and those credits need to be updated regularly. Each year there are a vast number of symposiums, conferences and workshops on a myriad of topics. Each one is allocated a set amount of credits towards continuing education. At these various symposiums, conferences and workshops, cardiologists have the opportunity to learn about the latest techniques available for treating a number of diseases. For example, there is a development towards stem cells being used to strengthen the hearts of patients with congestive heart failure. Or the physician could learn about the latest drugs released, such as angiotensin II receptor blockers. A physician would probably need to attend a number of these regularly in order to fill their quota of continuing education credits, but in this way, would not need to completely abandon their practice and patients and return to school to do so. Physicians and members of the group can often obtain their continuing education credits either at no cost, or at a lower rate per hour.

For clinicians in rural areas, it is often impractical to attend conferences that are far away. In addition to this, there are often no other clinicians available to care for their patients while they're gone. In this case, the internet has become a valuable resource for completing continuing education credits. A number of organizations facilitate continuing education online through coursework, online conferences and virtual lectures. In this way, a health care professional can obtain their continuing education credits from the comfort of their homes.

The system of continuing education is essential to the development of healthcare professionals. If this did not exist, the physician would be unable to remain fully apprised of any and all developments in their field, whether they are positive or negative. This lack of knowledge would finally result in improper, ineffectual, or possibly harmful care for patients. Essentially, the patients' quality of life depends largely on continuing education of physicians.

Made in the USA
Columbia, SC
06 May 2017